THE WITCH'S REMEDIES

BOTANICAL

MEDICINE

Over 75 healing

home

remedies for

various afflictions

Composed

by

a practicing hedge

witch

Welcome to the world of magical healing

When I was a child, my great grandmother used to tell

Me tales of fairies and enchanted forest creatures - the ones

Of the magical realm, whom I often saw in my dreams.

They would bring me wisdom of the knowledge, well-

Forgotten by our busy lives and filtered minds.

They told me that a physical affliction

Is nothing but a trapped energy that

Collects in a problematic area in the body as

A result of unresolved emotional stress and at

Times emotionally suppressed traumas

The fairies made me believe that most physical

Distress can be healed with a conscious choice knowing

That your unresolved emotions are the invisible cage

That keeps you in the world of mental darkness

Yet you're the only one who has the key

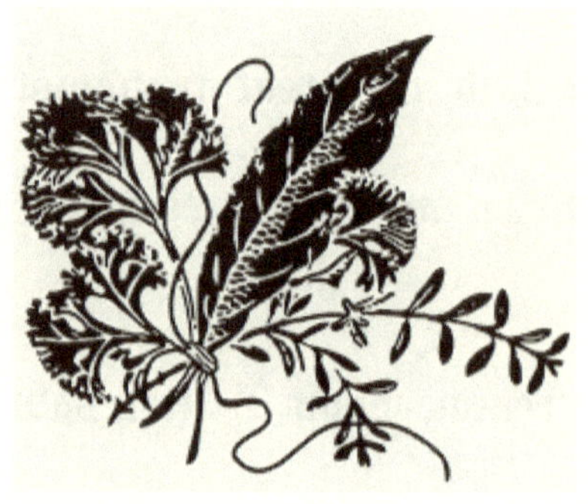

Life is thickly sown with thorns, and I know no other remedy than to pass quickly through them. The longer we dwell on our misfortunes, the greater is their power to harm us

Voltaire

BEAUTIFUL WITCHES

They are the beautiful creatures

Who know and understand

How to work with the energies

Around us

And use them for self or others'

Advantage and healing

They are great herbalists

Energy healers

Tarot readers

Mystics and philosophers of our time

They are the mavericks

Who make history

UNDERSTANDING HEALING

What causes your affliction

Can also heal you

For the antidote for a poisonous

Plant is derived

From the same plant

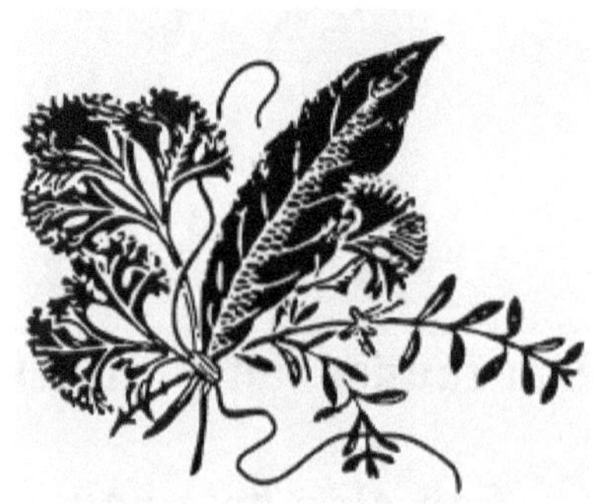

MORNING TENSION HEADACHE

(mental stress, over thinking)

Tension ache is provoked by

Tight neck muscle

Heat relaxes muscles

Drink a cup of hot tea or coffee

First thing to rid

Yourself of tension headache

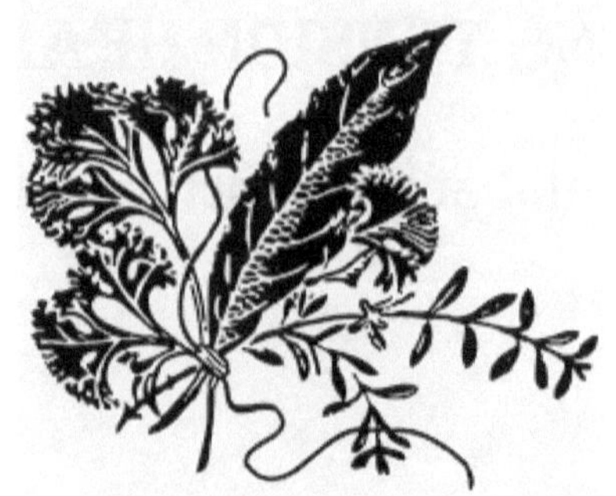

LOWER BACK PAIN

(guilt, shame, suppressed anger)

Applying ginger poultice onto

Lower back helps

Reduce pain in that area

Ginger works great for pulling

Inflammation from one's body

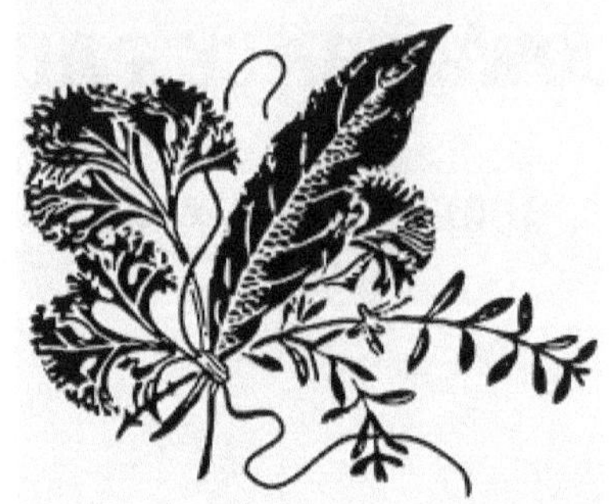

ACID REFLUX

(holding on to the past, sadness, grief)

Magnesium deficiency

Start taking magnesium twice

A day to help resolve it - no water or other liquid
consumption during meals

It washes down digestive enzymes

Instead try to drink a few

Minutes before each meal

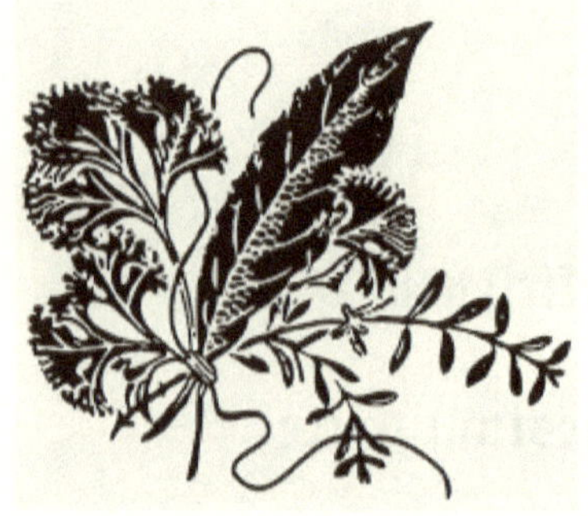

PSORIASIS

(shame, self-denial, disapproval)

Internal affliction

Not for topical remedy

Diet changes need be made

Avoid wheat, peanuts, oats,

Dairy and refined sugar

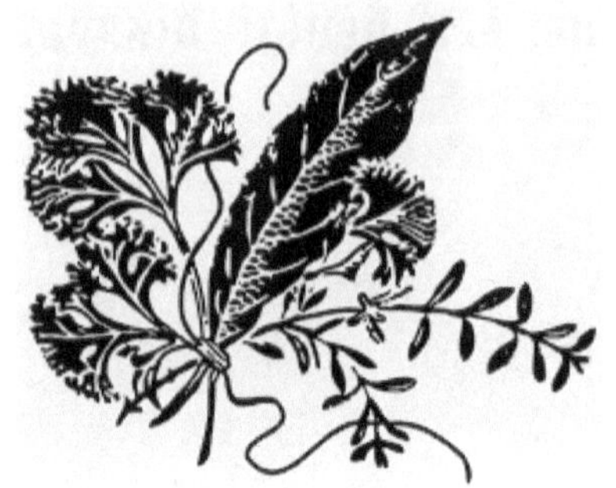

DIGESTION

(anger, anxiety, extreme sadness)

To help your digestion

Right before meal drink a cup

Of warm water with some juice from a freshly
squeezed lemon

In it

A lemon has the acid to aide pour digestion process

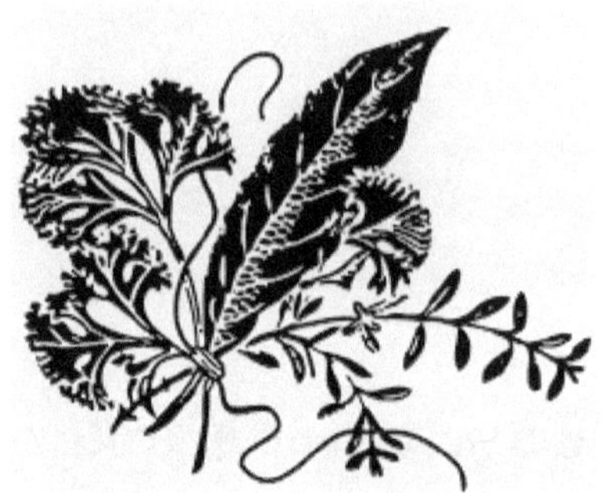

FIBROIDS, CYSTS

(depression, sexual discontent, unresolved
emotions connected to children or mother)

Castor oil topical application helps dissolve fibroid
and cysts on ovaries, as well as heal colon and
break up kidney stones and gallstones apply it on
abdomen or lower back where the distress dwells

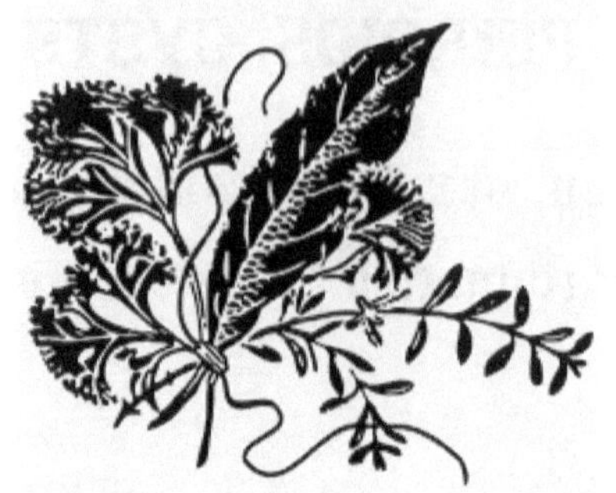

LIVER

(suppressed anger, depression, despair)

Between 1 and 3 A.M. toxins are

Released from the body and

Fresh new blood is made

Liver is active at this time of

Night

Liver stores unresolved anger

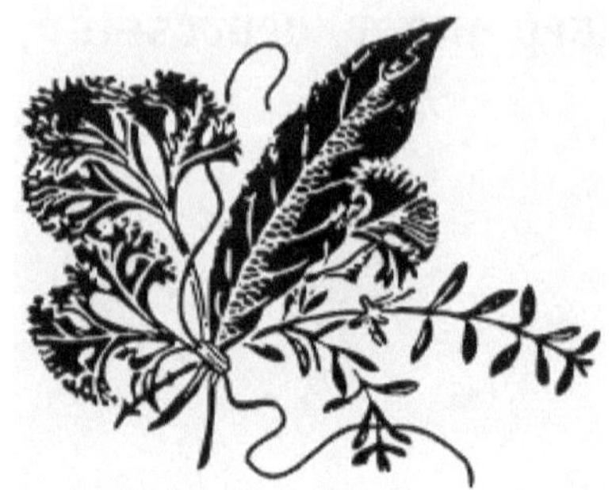

ESOPHAGUS AFFLICTION

(Unresolved anger, animosity, anxiety)

Remember that every physical affliction starts on emotional level for example

Esophagus is responsible for

Processing emotional traumas

Connected to unresolved emotions

With one's mother

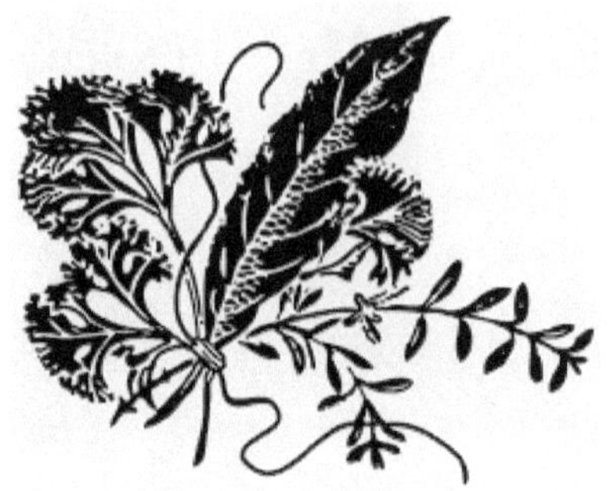

UNDERACTIVE THYROID

(inability for verbal expression, depression)

Cayenne pepper poultice placed

Onto throat

Revives thyroid gland

Thyroid imbalance has been linked

To iodine deficiency

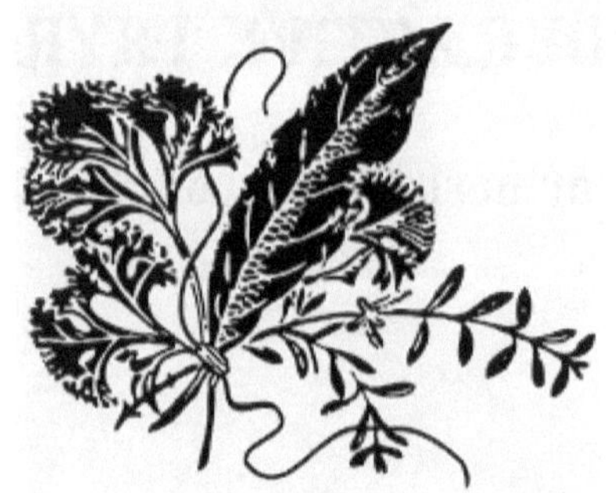

CANCER ONCOLOGY

(guilt, shame, self-rejection, suppressed anger)

Cancer loves refined sugar

Sugar deprives the body of oxygen making people with such malady feel very tired

Cancer also hates alkaline environment with no sugar it cannot survive in the body with a healthy liver

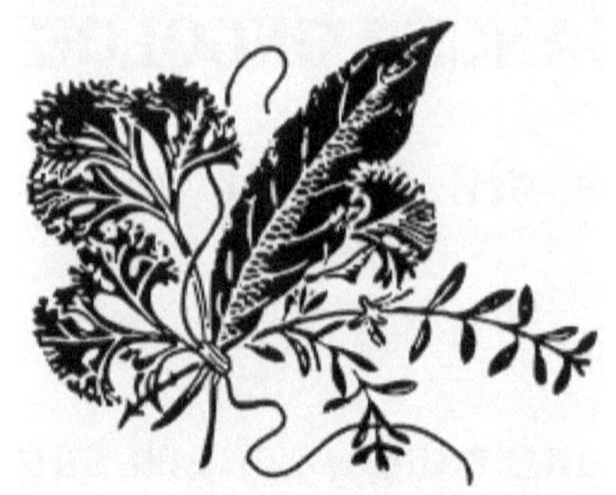

PERIPHERAL NEUROPATHY

(fear, worry, feeling unworthy)

With feet or hands numbness

Make a clear ceramic wrap with paper towel in it

Put some olive oil on paper towel and sprinkle half
a table spoon of powdered cayenne pepper

Wrap it around your hand or foot and leave it
overnight

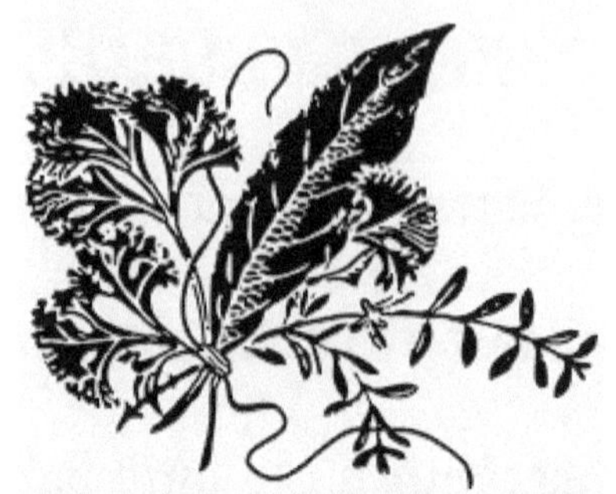

SEVERE COLD

(loss of vitality, depressed mood)

Using garlic as a powerful antibiotic is a great
remedy

Apply crushed raw garlic onto

Your bare feet in a sock overnight to break

Up chest congestion

Safe for small children as well

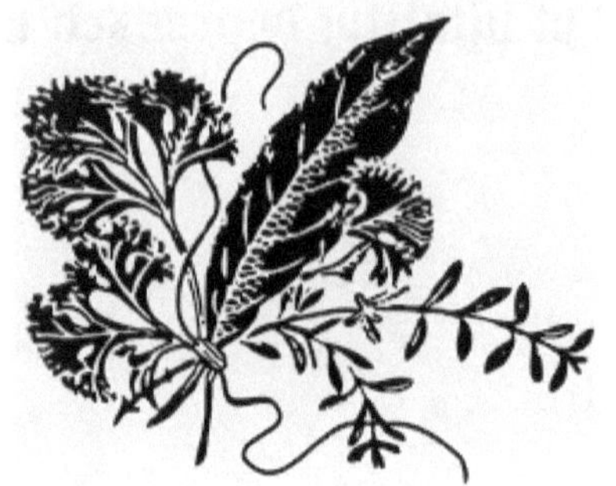

DIABETES

(unresolved anger in the past, fear, depression)

This affliction can be managed

Or in some cases treated

Fairly quickly by

Eliminating the carbohydrates in one's

Diet and avoiding refined sugar

As well as exercising

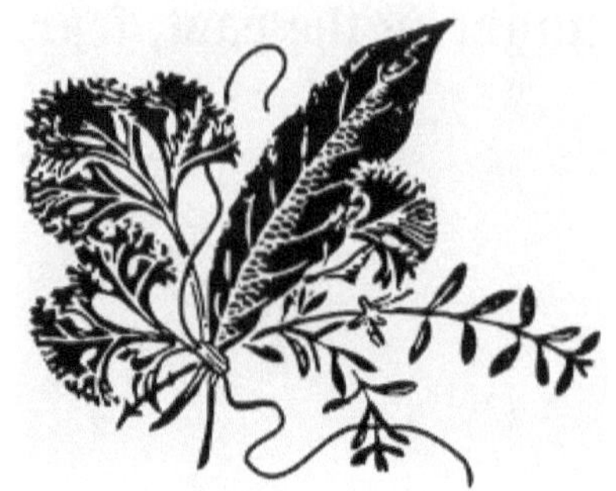

HIGH BLOOD PRESSURE

(suppressed anger, fear, worry)

Salt is very high in sodium

Your cell consists of potassium

Inside it

It also has sodium outside it

Salt enlarges the cell by pushing sodium into it
and that raises one's blood pressure

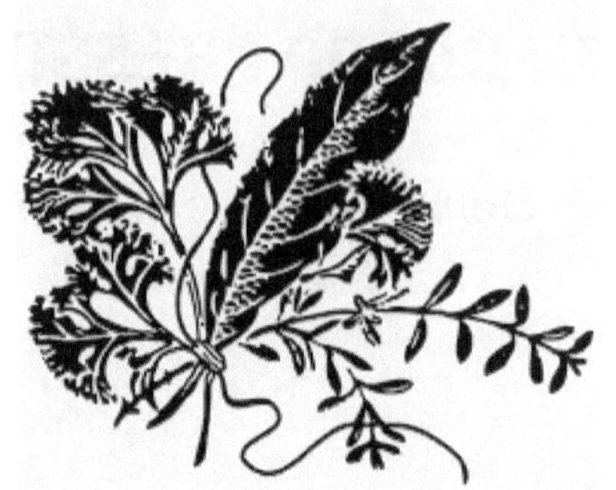

MORNING SICKNESS

(worry, anxiety, depression)

Feeling nauseous in the morning or during the day

Is a sign of magnesium deficiency

Unless you are with child

Start using magnesium to

Resolve the unpleasant malady

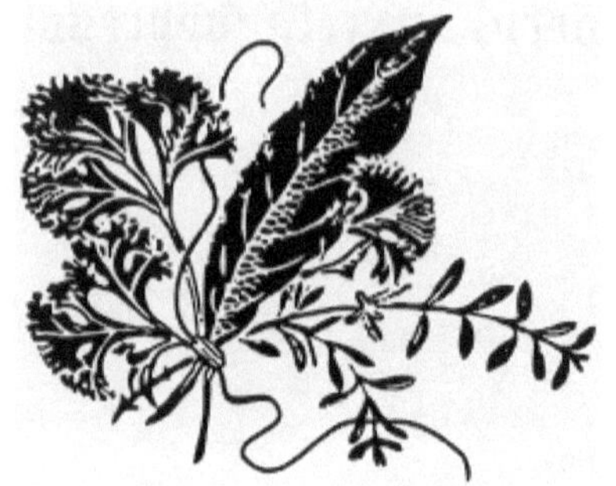

IMMUNE SYSTEM

(hostility, unresolved anger, self-denial)

Walking barefoot improves balance

Relieves physical pain and

Elevates mental distress

Improves sleep and eases anxiety

Regulates white blood cell count

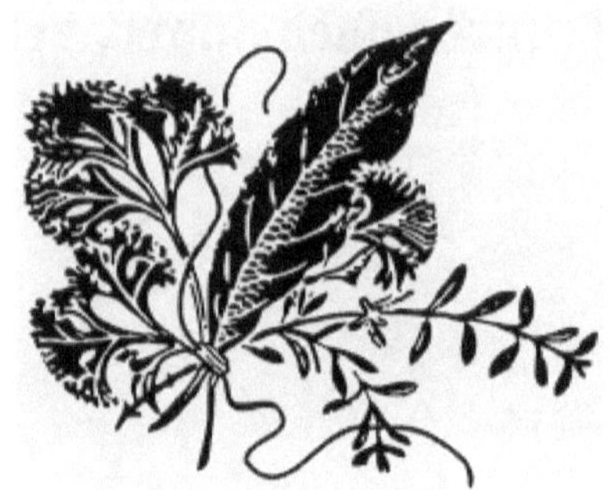

NIGHTMARES

(unresolved emotional stress, fear, anxiety)

Emotional stress in your waking life arises in a

form of a nightmare showing you the root

Of your emotional dilemma or

Unveiling a psychological ripple

Of your emotional state before it

Becomes a problem

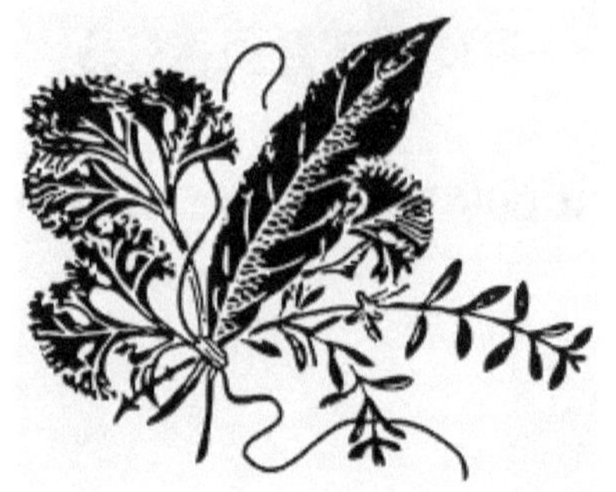

ACNE AND RELATED

(low self-worth, anxiety, fear to socialize)

Internal affliction

Topical treatment will not do much - drinking
fresh cabbage juice

Twice a day helps resolve it

By making skin visibly lighter

And by protecting skin cells from

Radical damage

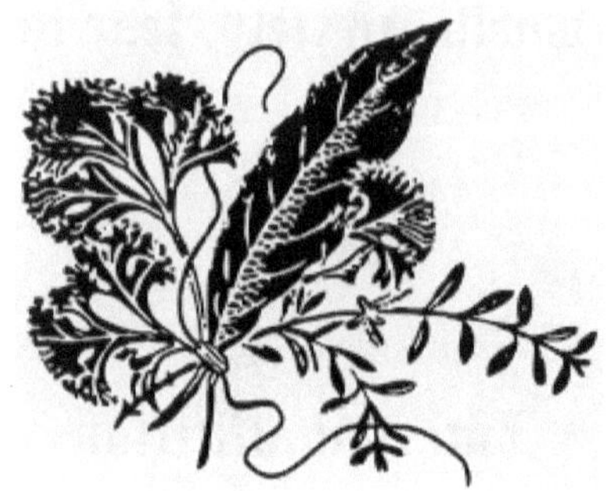

INTESTINAL TRACT

(anger, anxiety, extreme sadness)

Freshly made juice from pineapple and cucumber

detoxifies colon by removing excess waste from

Intestinal tract

For pineapples contain enzymes

To deliver protein to help your body

Reduce inflammation

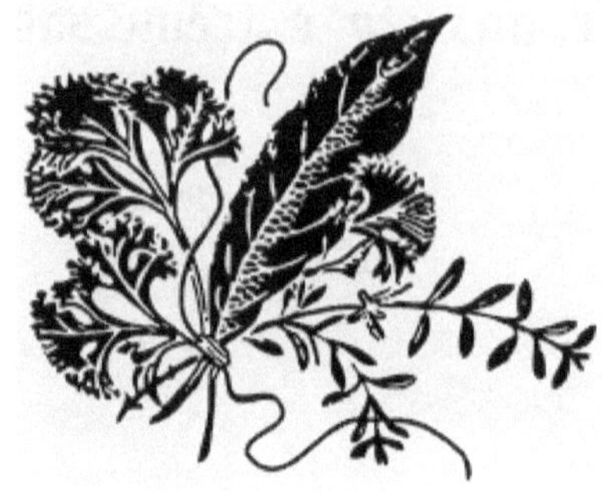

WOUNDS AND BURNS

(short-lived stress, self-blame, fear)

Aloe Vera plant's natural gel is great for healing wounds

Burns and scratches by speeding up

Recovery process with its anti-bacterial and anti-inflammatory

properties

Do not apply on open wounds

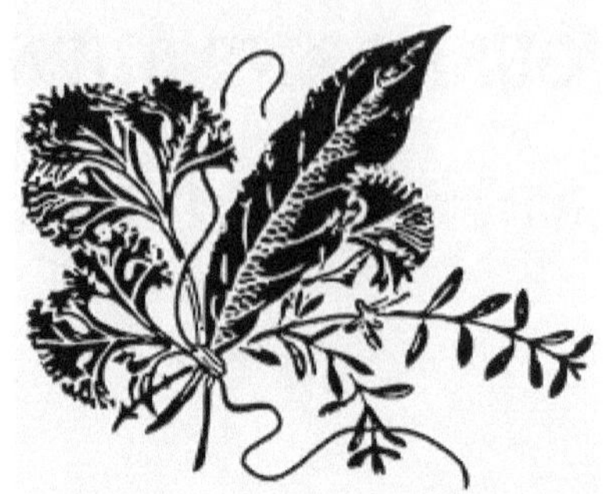

PULLED MUSCLE

(inability to cope with stress, insecurity)

Topical treatment with comfrey

Ointment does well for

Pulled muscles and ligaments

As well as sprains and

Osteoarthritis

Topical application only

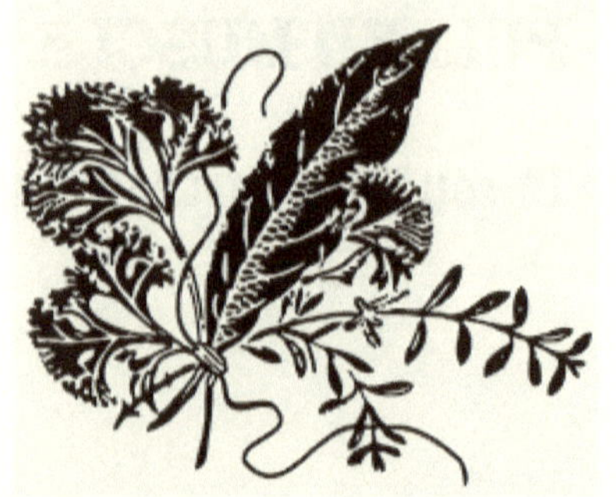

UPSET STOMACH

(inability to process emotions, fear, sorrow)

Making a ginger tea helps

Settle the stomach and eliminate

Nausea

Ginger is great for reducing

Inflammation and

Warming the body up internally

If needed

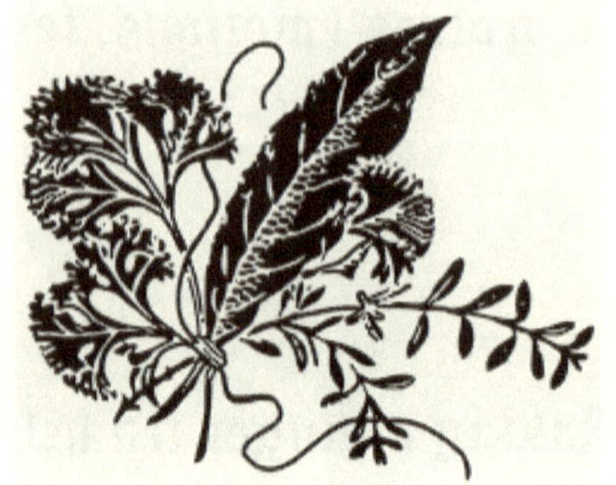

SPRAINED ANKLE

(inner insecurity, fear of one's future)

Fresh cabbage leaves wrapped

Around one's ankle

Are great for bruised and sprained

Ankles

Also when breastfeeding to reduce

Pain and engorgement

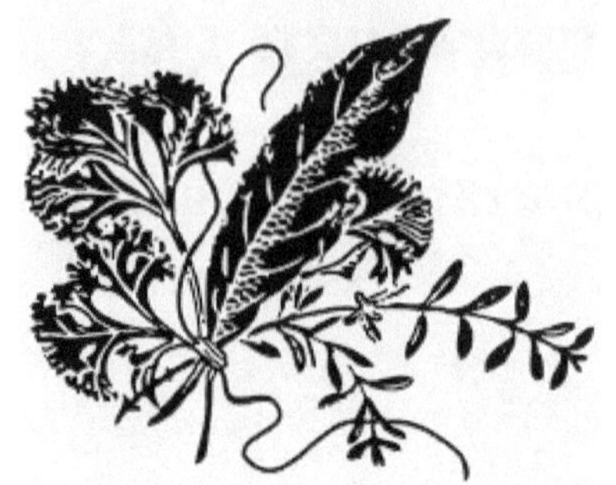

MENTAL AFFLICTION

(unresolved fear, anger, worry, self-denial)

Burning bay leaves helps ease

One's anxiety and depression

Bay leaves' smoke produces linalool

Which affects one's serotonin receptor

Bay leaf incense helps

Combat insomnia as well

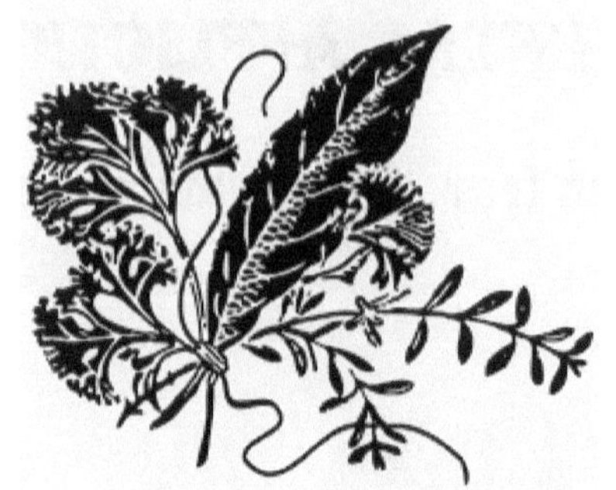

SKIN BLEMISHES

(self-denial, insecurity, non-acceptance, fear)

Use Aloe Vera plant's natural gel as a facial
topical application

To cleanse and tighten skin

It helps clear up blemishes as well as eases
sunburn on skin

It is a natural moisturizer

Having anti-aging properties

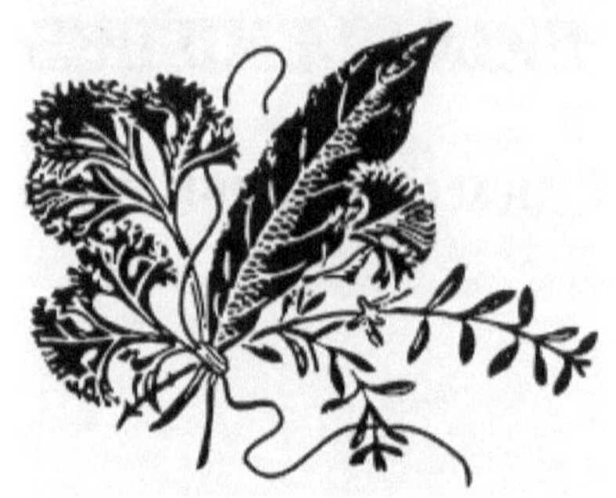

CONSTIPATION

(suppressed anger, guilt, inability to express)

Yellow dragon fruit happens

To be a natural laxative and is

Very helpful when it comes to these

Uncomfortable matters

The fruit is very rich in fiber

And that helps the colon move waste

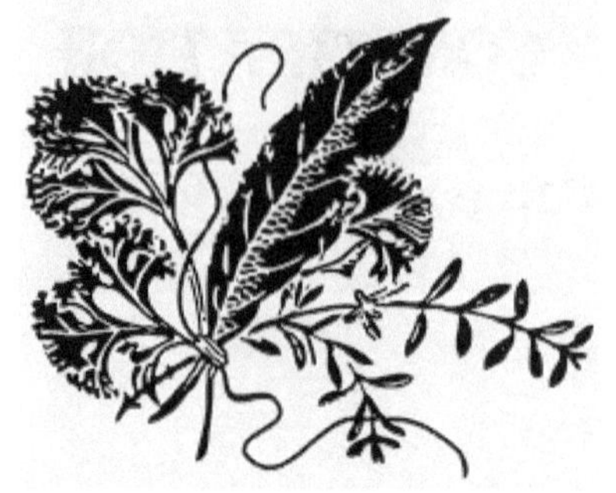

SWOLLEN EYES

(fear to face truth, guilt, self-rejection)

Raw potato poultice is

Great for tissue inflammation

Including the one of swollen eyes

Red eyes and injured eyes

It also helps with ingrown toe nails

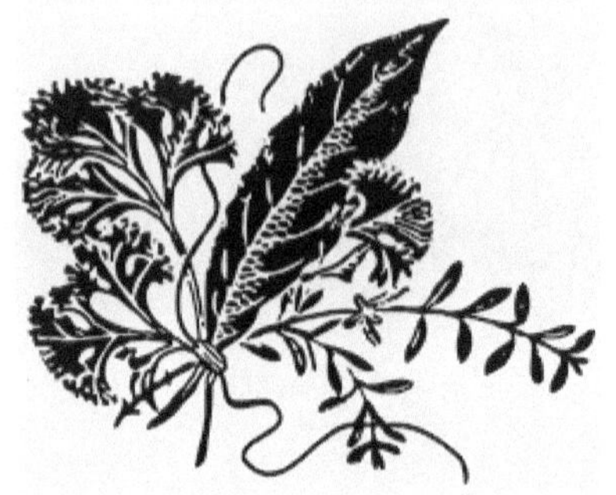

STAPHYLOCOCCUS (STAPH)

(unresolved anger, inability to forgive)

Goldenseal root is known

To be one of the best herbs to assist with

This unpleasant affliction

The root kills the infection by

Inhibiting the growth of gram-positive

Bacteria

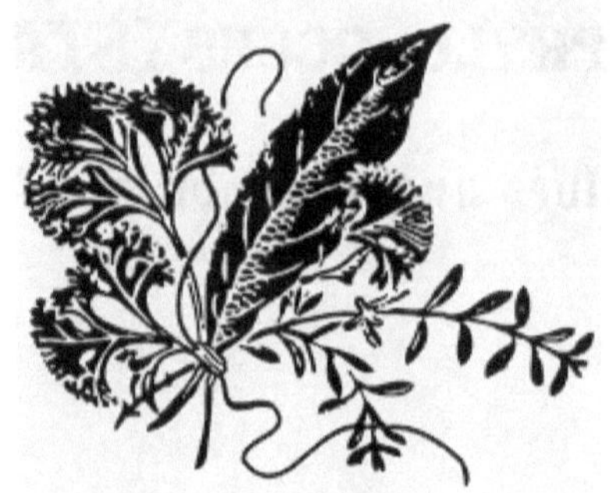

KIDNEY STONES

(suppressed anger, depression, despair)

Drinking pure organic lemon juice helps one rid of
this nuisance

By dislodging the stones

For lemons contain citric acid which can break
down kidney stones

Also preventing excess calcium

From forming

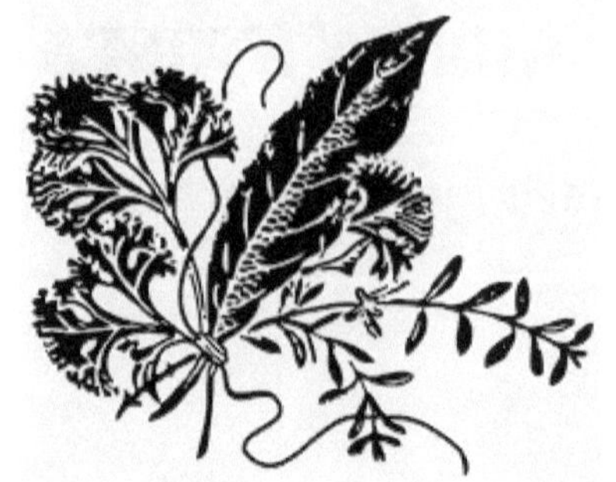

MENOPAUSE DISCOMFORT

(depression, living in the past)

Hormonal imbalance can be

Helped with maintaining organic

Diet and taking

Vitamins such as b6 b9 and b12

Liver detox is a must

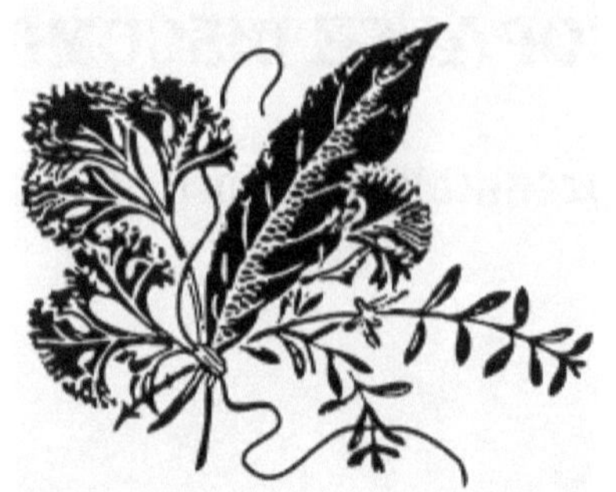

HEART PALPITATIONS

(anxiety, fear, panic in thought)

Slowly and deeply inhaling and exhaling

Three times in a row

Immediately reinstates the heart

Rate and brings one back

To resting heart rate

Eliminate worry for all is temporary

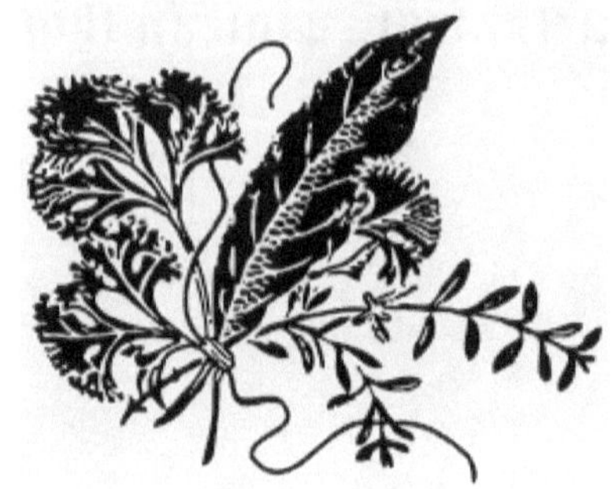

LYMPHATIC SYSTEM

(unresolved negative emotions, mental chaos)

Our lymphatic system is also known to be a drainage system that

Processes and releases all sorts

Of emotional mental and physical waste

It can easily become energetically

Blocked by various unresolved emotions

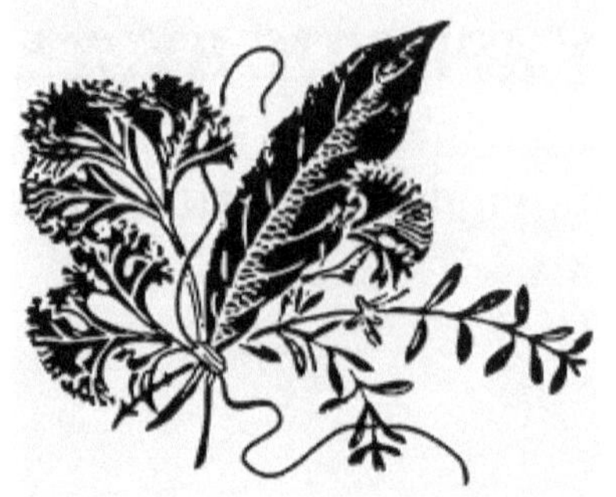

BLOCKED ARTERIES

(self-rejection, criticism, shame, guilt)

A pinch of fresh powdered

Cayenne pepper with half a glass

Of water is one of the best

Known blood thinners out there

It also helps lower blood pressure

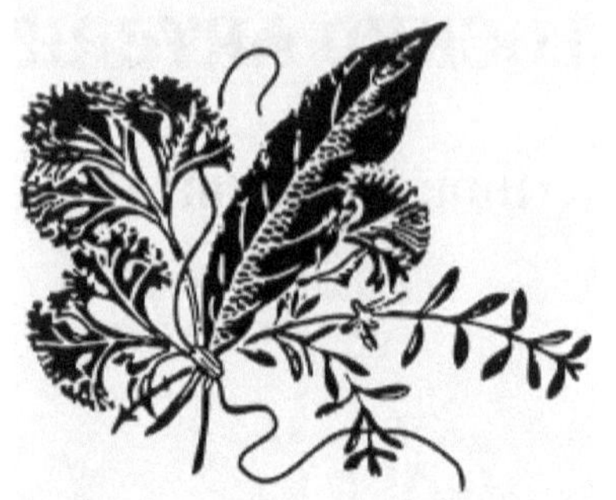

DIAPER RASH

(even little angels can experience emotional stress)

A paste with baking soda and

Water helps resolve this

Uncomfortable dilemma

For baking soda is great at reducing skin
inflammation and

Irritation

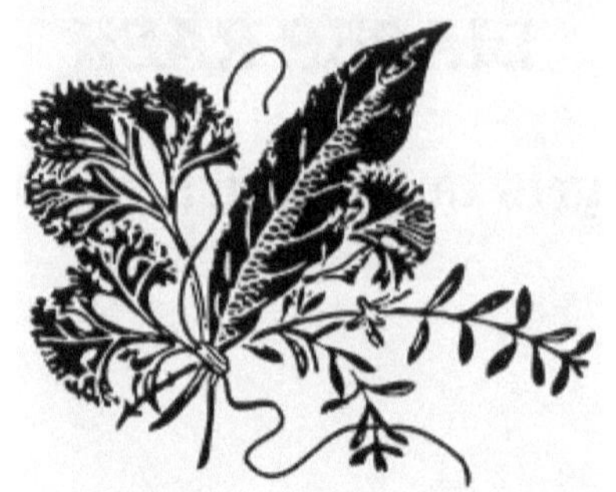

ABSCESSED TOOTH

(inability to verbally express oneself, weakened
self-esteem)

Raw onion can be applied to an abscessed tooth or
a boil

It is great at pulling infection out of the body

Onion juice with honey can be

Used as a lovely cold remedy

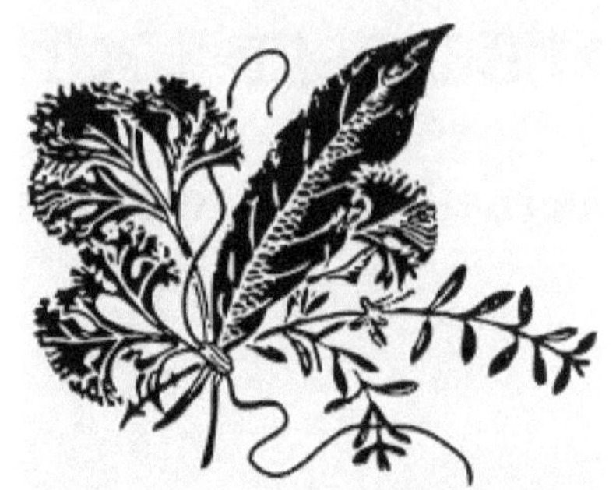

LONG-REPRESSED SHOCK

(suppressed emotional trauma, fear)

Star of Bethlehem flowers help

Gradually recover from long-repressed

Emotional trauma along with

Psychosomatic disorder which may

Have derived from the initial shock

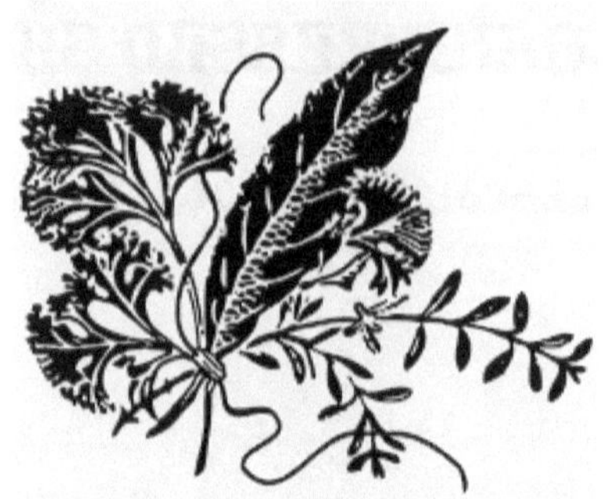

CHEST CONGESTION

(feeling unloved, self-criticism, depression)

Raw crushed onion wrapped

Around the feet with socks on

And worn overnight is great for

Healing chest congestion and head colds

Along with other respiratory distress

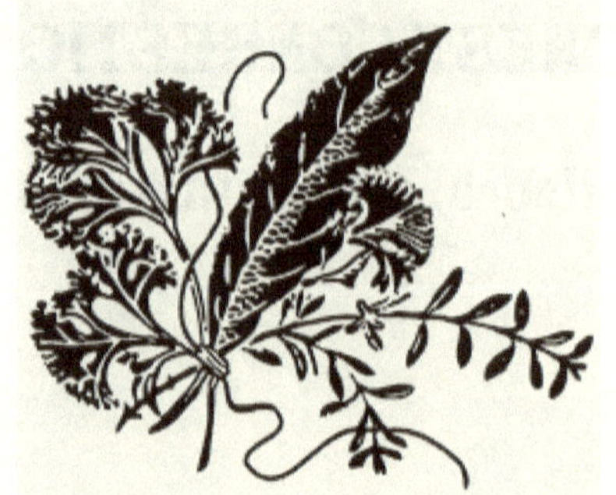

SUDDEN STRESS AND UPSET

(unwillingness to change, anxiety, fear)

Rescue remedy is needed made from 5 flower
combination

Cherry Plum, Clematis, Impatiens,

Rock Rose, Star of Bethlehem

Put 4 drops in a glass of water and

Sip throughout the day

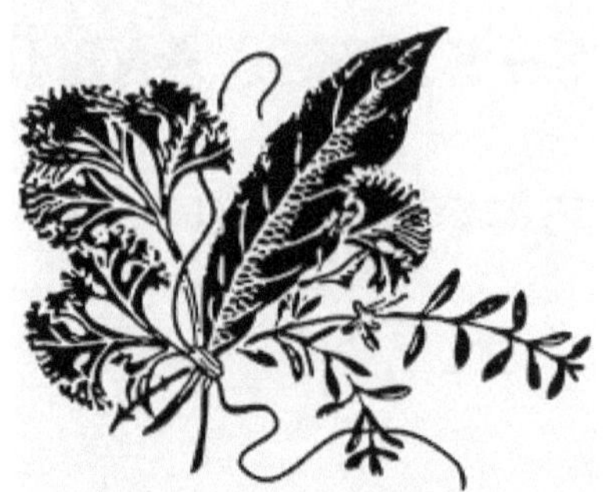

EARWAX

(disconnection, apathy, emotional withdrawal)

One drop of warmed almond oil

Put into the ear with a small dropper

Usually does the trick

By softening the wax inside the ear

And making it easier to remove

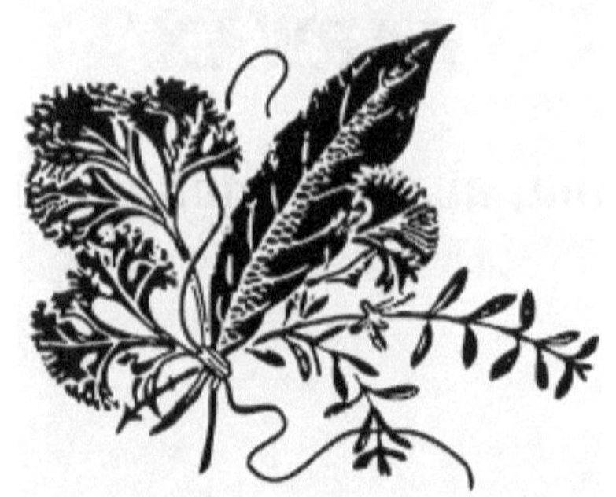

BAD BREATH

(self-blame, self-criticism, anger)

Chewing fresh coriander seeds or

Cilantro after meals

Help resolve bad breath quickly

The seeds help elevate strong food

Odours that may provoke bad breath

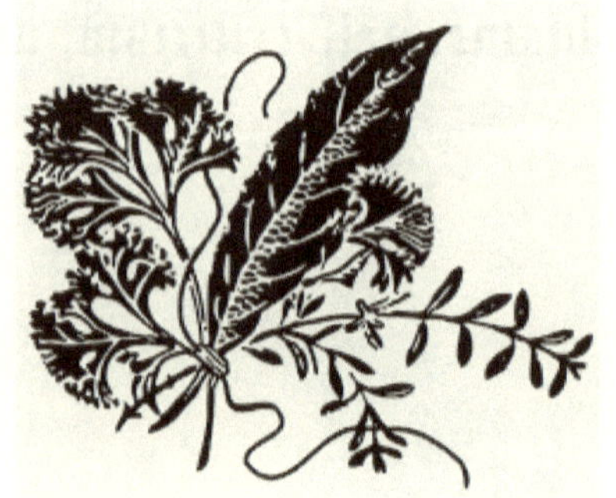

STOMACH ULCER

(extreme sadness, loss of control, depression)

Cayenne pepper comes very handy when it comes to
ulcers

¼ teaspoon of powdered pepper mixed

With a small glass of water

Cayenne pepper constricts open blood

Vessels thus helping resolve such issue

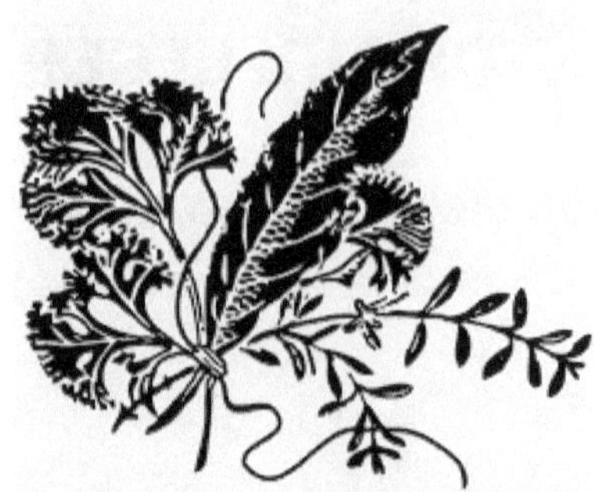

BLEEDING WOUND

(insecurity, fear, feeling of not being grounded)

Cayenne pepper saves the day again

Just quickly apply the powder

Onto the bleeding cut or wound

It may sting a bit but it

Will stop the bleeding

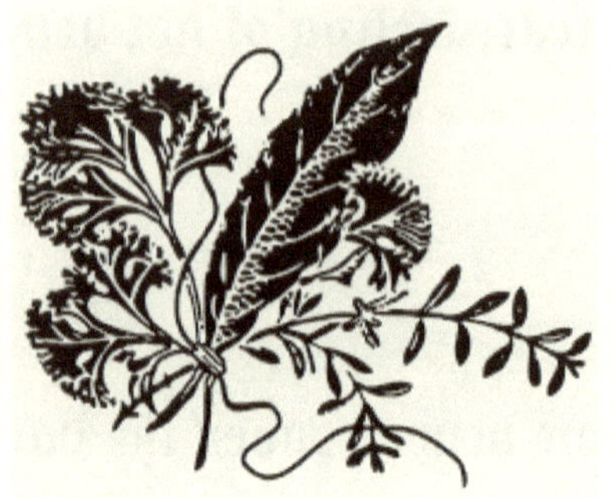

EXCESSIVE PHLEGM

(suppressed speech, inability to verbally express
oneself)

Elder flower tincture is

Very useful when it comes to

Trying to rid of phlegm after

A bad cold or other respiratory distress

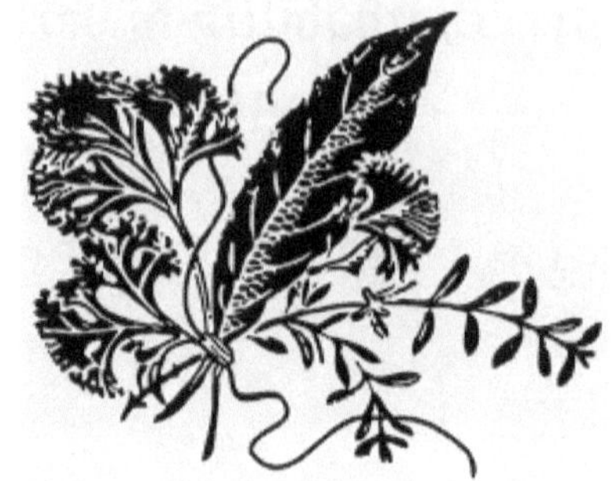

FALLING HAIR

(energy loss, fear, anxiety, internal fatigue)

Use the decoction with the root

Of stinging Nettle to rinse

Your hair with

Also helps with

dandruff problem

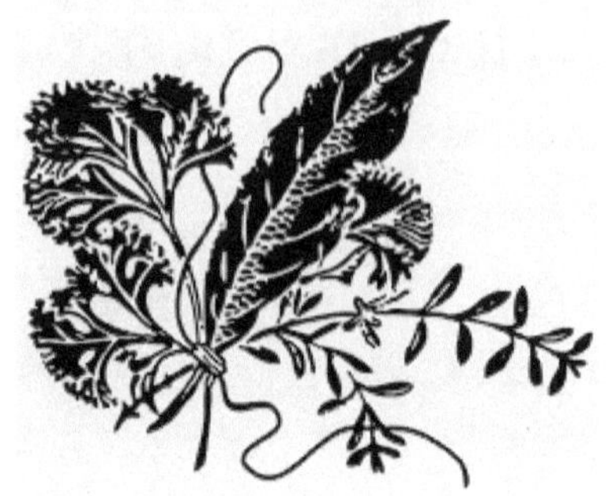

ASTHMA

(loos of control, fear, suppressed anger)

This affliction is primarily caused

By phlegm produced by

Weakened spleen and kidneys

Steam inhalation from chamomile and

Ecalyptus eases panic and helps

Open the airways

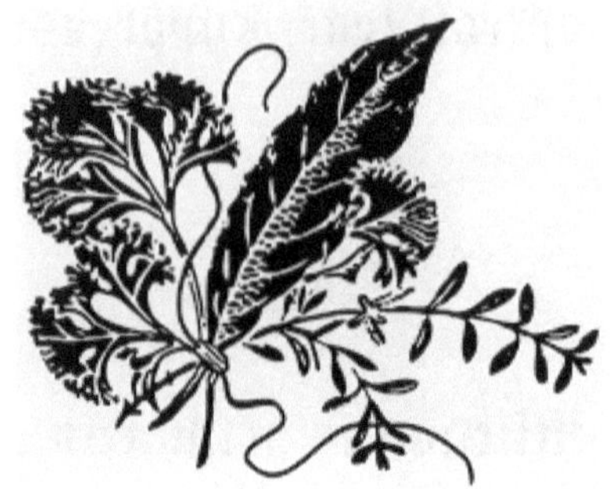

GALLSTONES

(suppressed sadness, guilt, depression)

Castor oil applied on the distressed

Area helps dissolve them

As well as a tea blend with balmony, dandelion
leaves, stone root and fringetree bark taken

Twice a day resolve the issue within

Several months

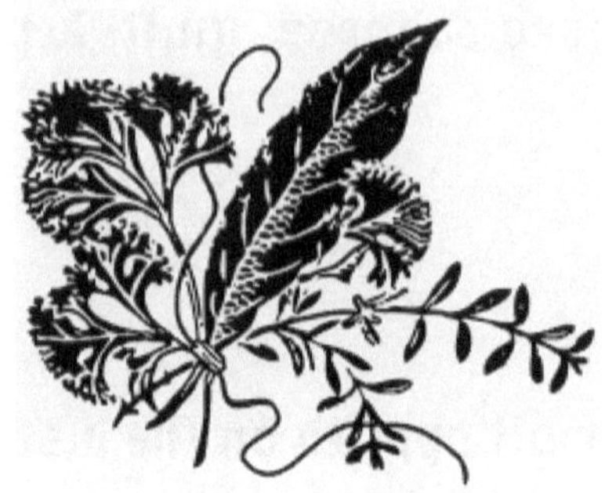

TRAVEL SICKNESS

(fear of the future, loss of control, mental chaos)

When you travel and you feel

Nausea coming up,

Chew on fresh ginger or sip ginger tea

This will elevate the

symptoms

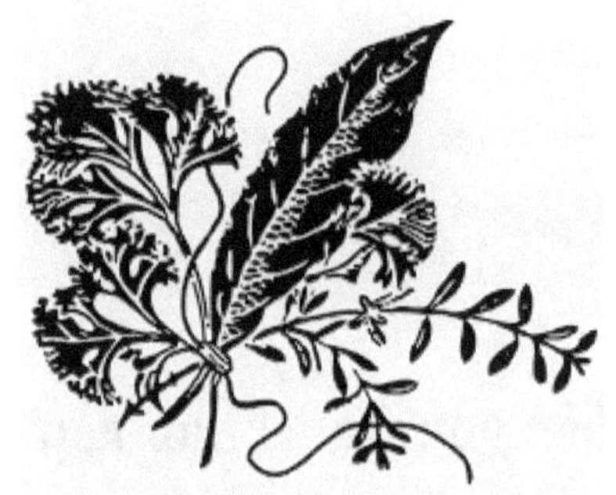

MULTIPLE SCLEROSIS

(fear, loss of identity, unresolved emotional trauma)

Diet change is a must. Foods that

Contain gamma-linoleic acid along

With vitamins of b3, b6 and b12

Vitami c and e as well as

Minerals and magnesium rich foods

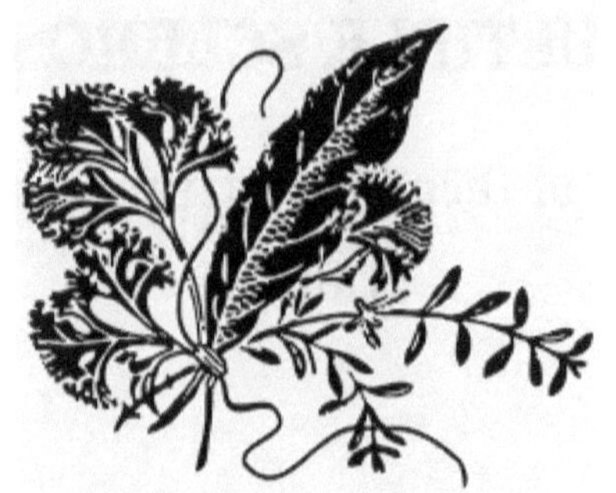

EPILEPSY

(fear, depression, buried sadness)

Foods rich in magnesium calcium

And zinc may reduce the attack

Frequency as well as vitamins b5 and b6

Herbal tea with vervain and valerian

May help prevent attacks

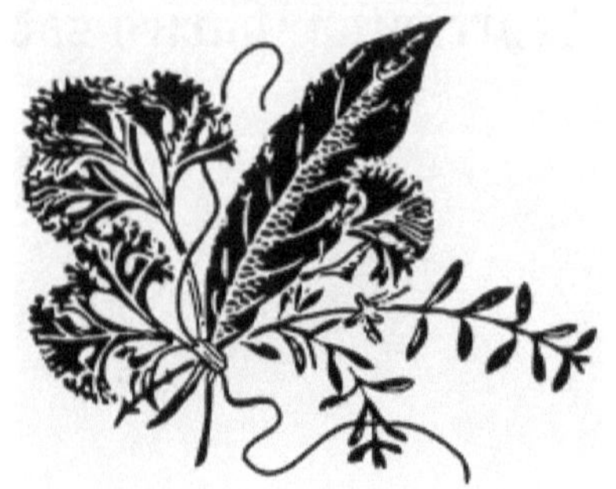

WARTS

(self-criticism, shame, guilt, fear)

Rubbing fresh lemon onto

The wart will dry and lighten the skin

Diminishing the appearance of it

Castor oil mixed with baking soda

Paste also helps solve the problem

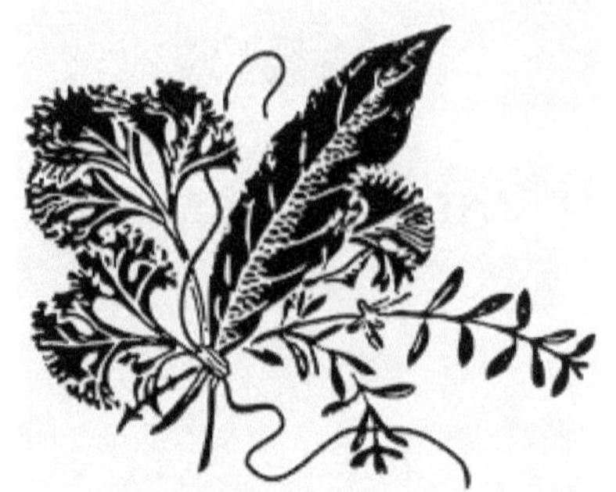

COLD SORE

(self-criticism, shame, self-rejection)

Fresh lemon comes in handy again

Rubbing lemon on the cold sore

Helps dry it up

St. John's wort tincture may be

Applied to prevent further growth

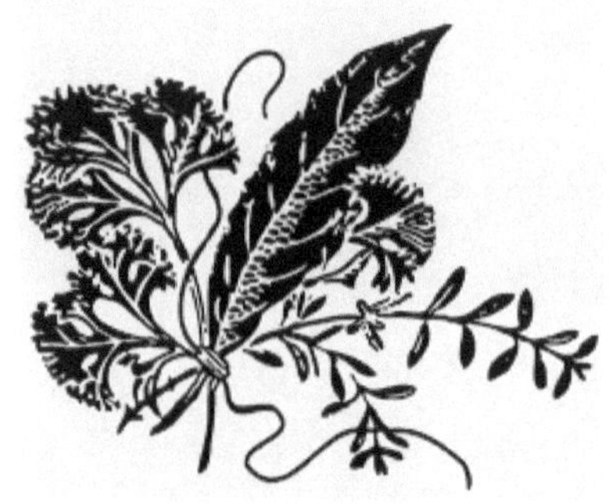

BLACK EYE

(short-term stress, inability to accept current events)

A cooled infusion from fresh

Lavender leaves may be applied

Under the eye to help healing it

Followed by arnica gel

Topical application

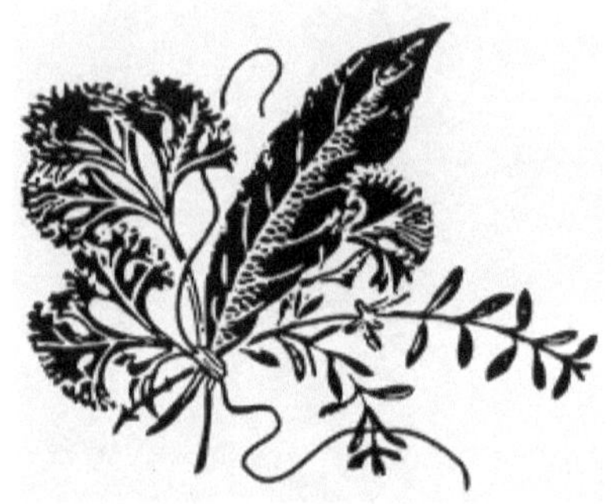

STYE

(inability to see things for what they are, self-denial)

A poultice from warmed bread

Applied onto the eye helps

Bring out the infection

Also a raw potato slice topical

Application may be done for the same purpose

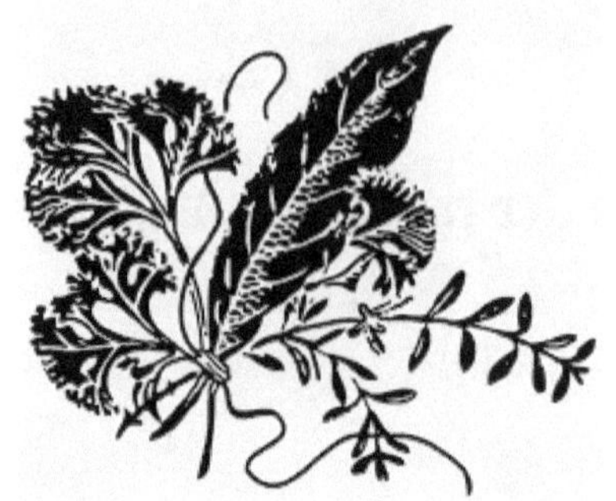

HAY FEVER

(short-term stress, fear of new experiences)

Eating fresh garlic with or

Before your meals helps boost

The immune system and make

The allergic reaction

dissipate quicker

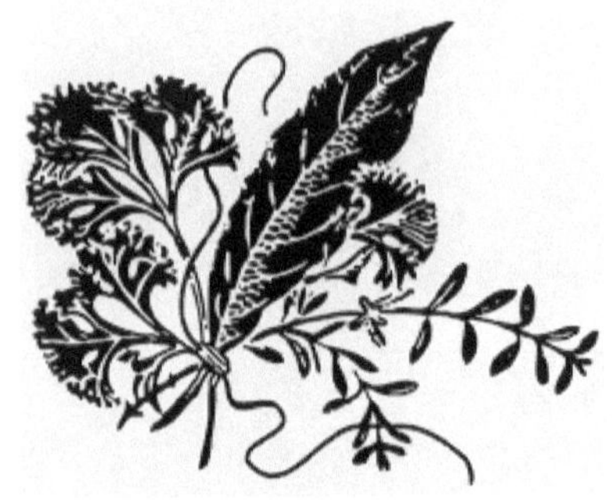

BRONCHITIS

(inability to deal with responsibilities, self-blame
and rejection)

Hoeny and lemon taken with hot tea helps ease the
cough and fight off the infection

A poultice with raw onion wrapped

Around the feet and

left overnight

Works as a chest decongestant

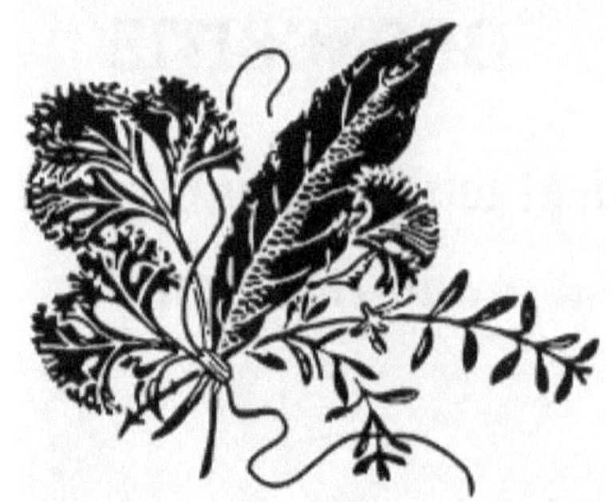

HICCUPS

(fear to face reality, unacceptance of current truth)

Sucking on a fresh lemon

Usually stops the hiccups fairly

Quickly

It needs be mentioned to keep

A fresh lemon handy

at all times

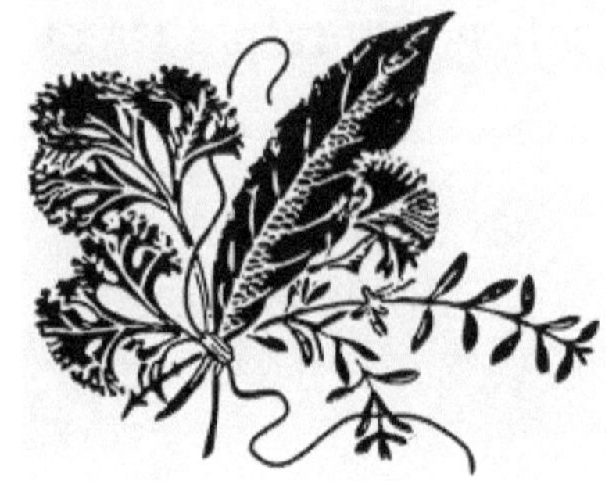

LOW BLOOD PRESSURE

(suppressed self-expression, fear of the unknown)

Tea made with hawthorn tops

May be helpful

Along with ginger and rosemary

To stimulate blood circulation

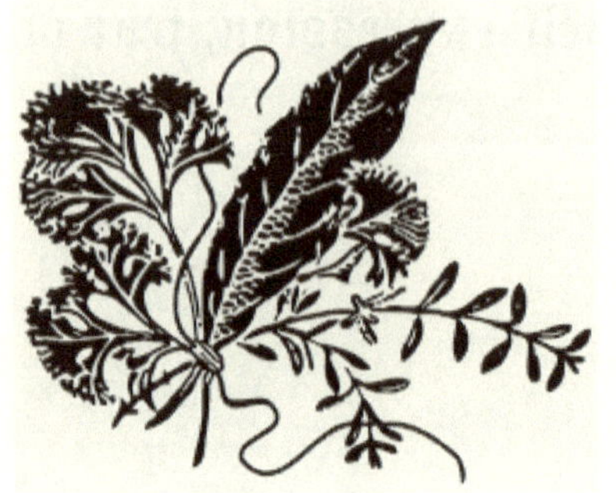

BREASTFEEDING

(short-term emotional stress, fear, self-criticism)

When it comes to breastfeeding and

Brest engorgement

Putting fresh cabbage leaves in

Your bra between feedings

solves the problem

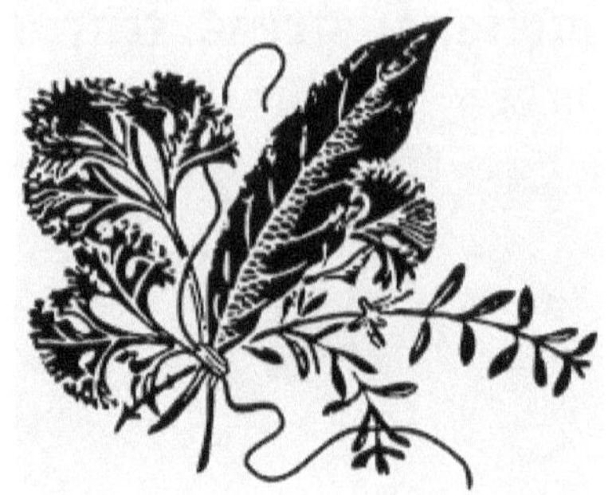

HIGH BLOOD PRESSURE

(suppressed anger, fear, past regrets)

Mineral deficiency

Is one of the causes

Use the foods rich in magnesium

Along with keeping Celtic salt

In your kitchen and adding it

To your food

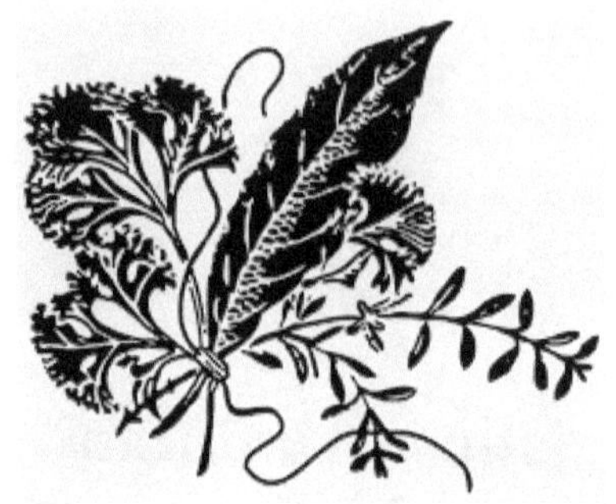

BREAST CYSTS

(self-denial, fear, rejection of womanhood)

A topical application of castor oil

Helps dissolve the cysts

And lumps on the breast

Some studies show it has a potential to diminish
and dissipate breast lumps connected to cancer

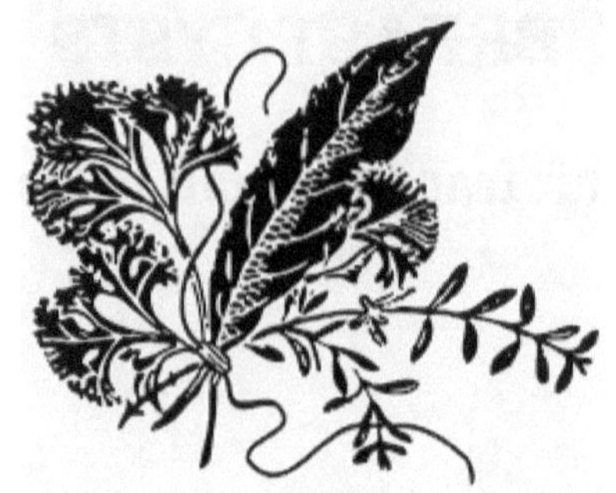

PARASITES

(giving away personal power, letting others control you)

Eating raw pumpkin seeds usually solves the problem quickly

Eating raw galic is helpful

Can help animals with parasites as well by crushing ¼ teaspoon of raw seeds in their food

Resolves mostly within 2-3 days

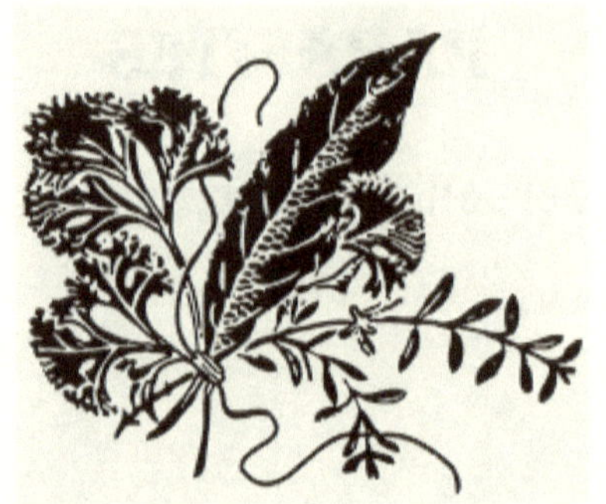

ERECTAL DYSFUNCTION

(damaged self-worth, loss of self-confidence)

Emotional problem

Needs to heal the root of the affliction

By restoring a good opinion about thyself

In the meantime use

A pinch of sandalwood back in a small glass

Of water to help the physical matter to rise

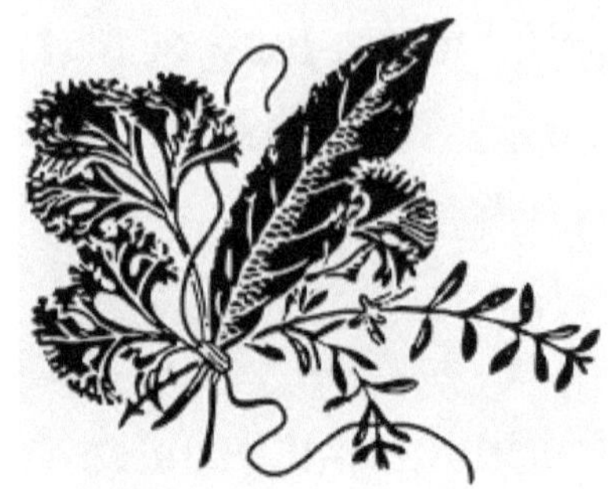

DANDRUFF

(insecurity, low-self-esteem, anxiety)

Rubbing rosemary oil onto

The dry scalp helps resolve

The dry hair problem

Mineral deficiency

Consuming dark green leafy greens

Helps maintain

healthy hair

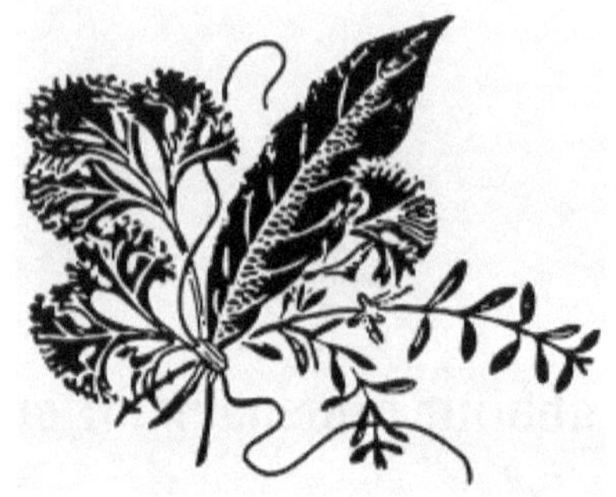

DRY SKIN

(distorted self-image, fear of public engagement)

Apply a paste made with sandalwood

Bark powder and yogurt onto

The problematic skin area

Once a week to

resolve the issue

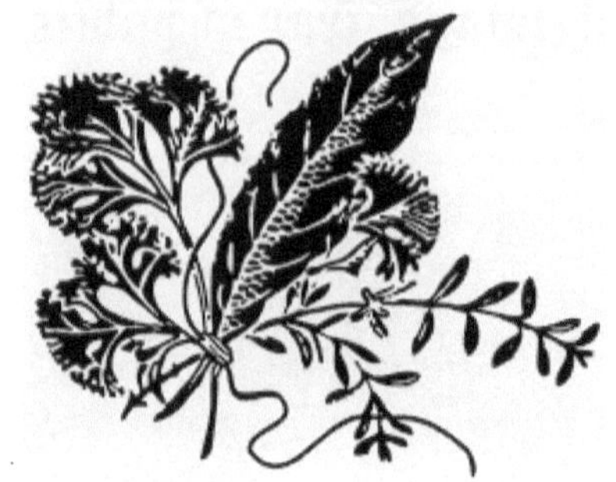

LIVER DISTRESS

(suppressed anger, inability to forgive, depression)

A good time for the liver detox

Which consists of drinking lots of

Water with lemon

Or diluted lemon juice if you wish

And avoiding all refined sugar

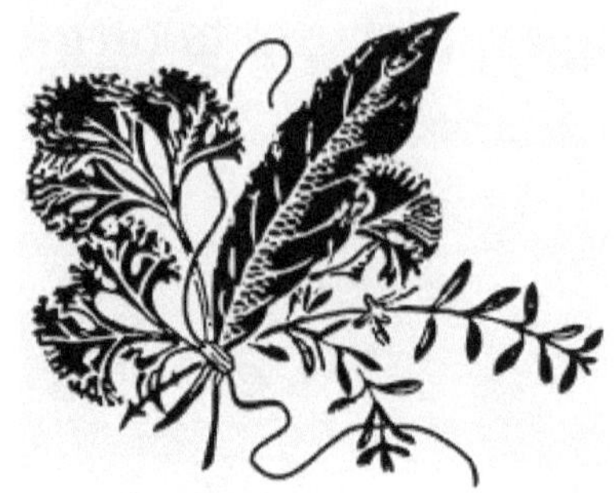

VARICOSE ULCERS

(internal chaos, self-denial, inability to accept love)

Make a poultice with powdered comfrey

Root and water

And apply onto the distressed area

And other stubborn scars and wounds

The paste also helps with bleeding hemorrhoids

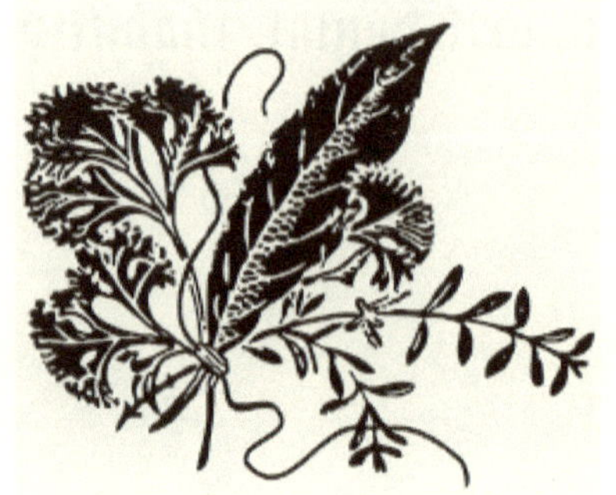

TIRED BRAIN

(emotional stress overload, self-disapproval)

Extreme fatigue can cause the brain feeling very
tired and sleepy

Three things that can help are

Intermittent diet

Finishing a hot shower with a cold one

Running up the hill exercise

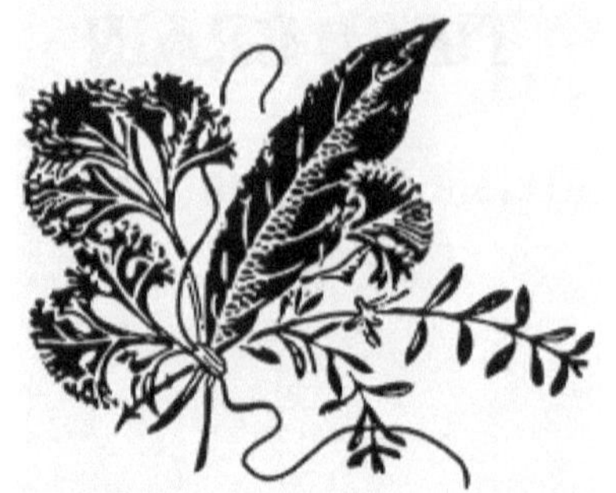

INFERTILITY (WOMAN)

(fear, self-blame, unresolved emotions with one's mother)

Such affliction is associated with emotional stress creating a hormonal

Imbalance

Eat oats as often as possible

They help manage general stress Unresolved emotional trauma is the main cause

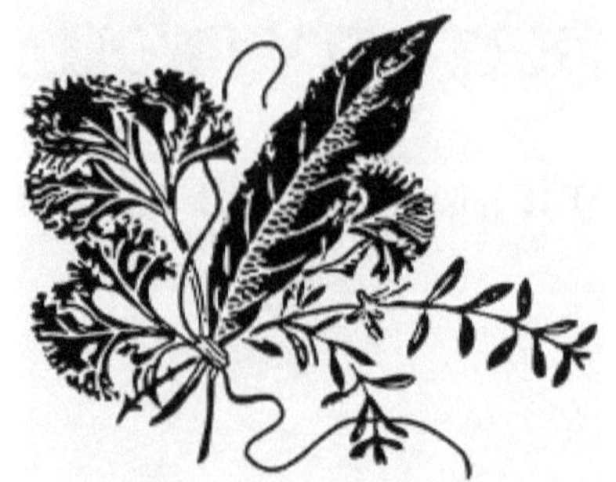

INSOMNIA DUE TO NERVES

(inability to accept the present, fear, anxiety)

Valerian root taken as in tincture

Or tea helps with insomnia and

The nervousness

Also rescue remedy comes in handy

When you feel the symptoms coming on

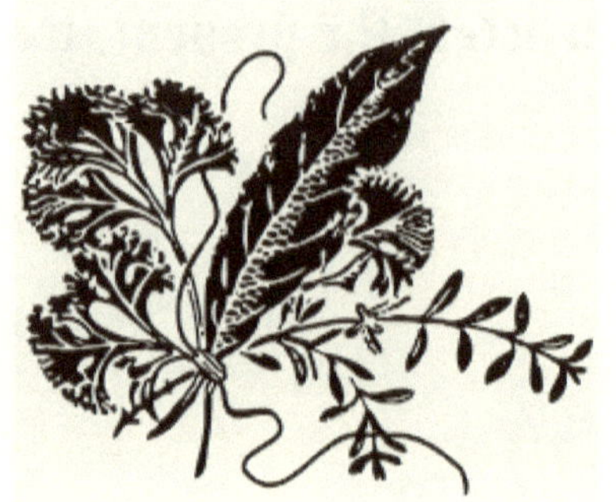

SLUGGISH LIBIDO

(self-esteem, compromised self-confidence)

A fenugreek tea traditionally

Can be used as an aphrodisiac for it

Stimulates uterus

Also can be used for male impotence

Avoid when pregnant

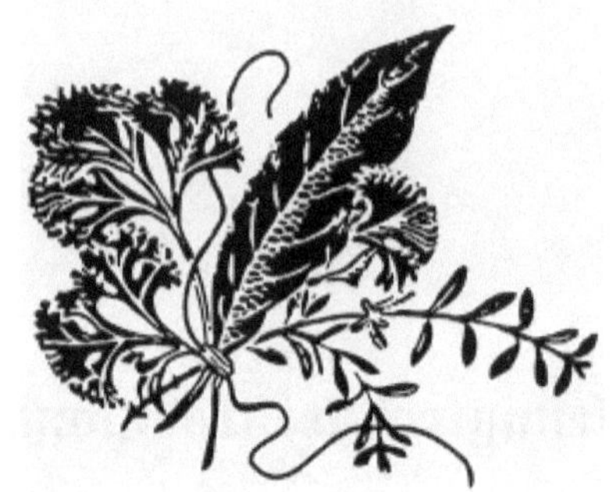

CHRONIC COUGH

(suppressed sadness, unspoken truth,
disappointment)

To assist with chronic coughs such as

Whooping cough tuberculosis asthma

And bronchitis use mullein

Comes in tinctures and infusions

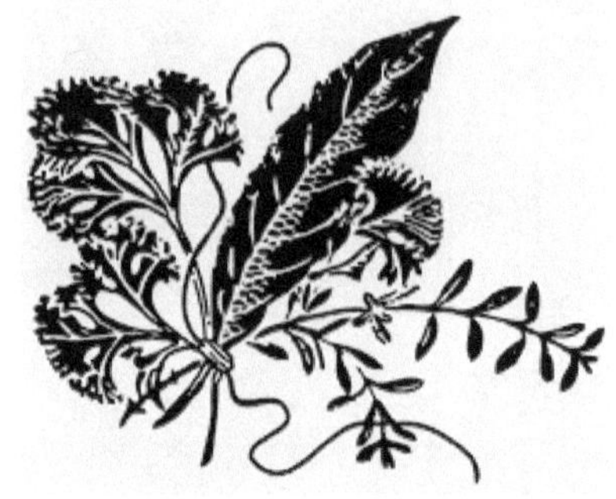

ENDOMETRIOSIS

(unresolved emotions with one's mother, loss of
self-worth, fear)

Castor oil poultice is to be

Applied on the lower abdomen to

Help eliminate excess tissues and

Toxins inside the body

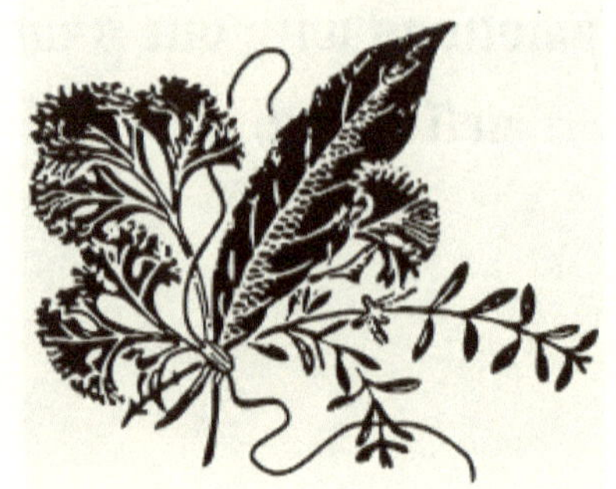

PROSTATE

(weakened sense of self-worth and self-esteem,
unresolved emotions with one's father)

Watercress leaves should be part

Of ongoing diet as well as

Pumpkin seeds tonic is a great one

To help solve the issue

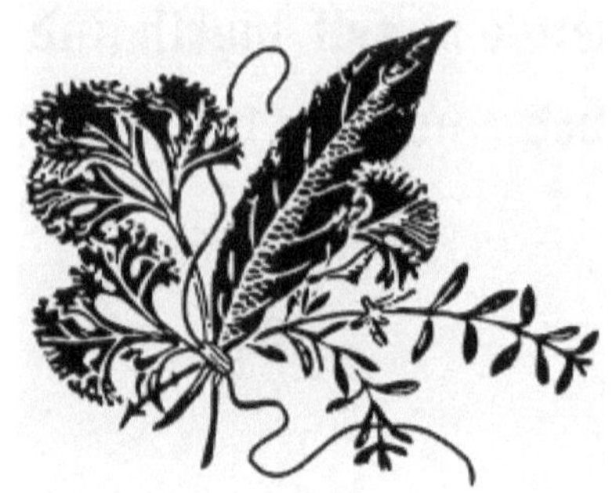

OBESITY

(damaged self-image, self-worth, fear, sadness)

A glass of fresh grapefruit juice

Drunk every morning helps

Cleanse the body break down fats and suppress
appetite

Use caution when taking medication

For grapefruit can overpower it

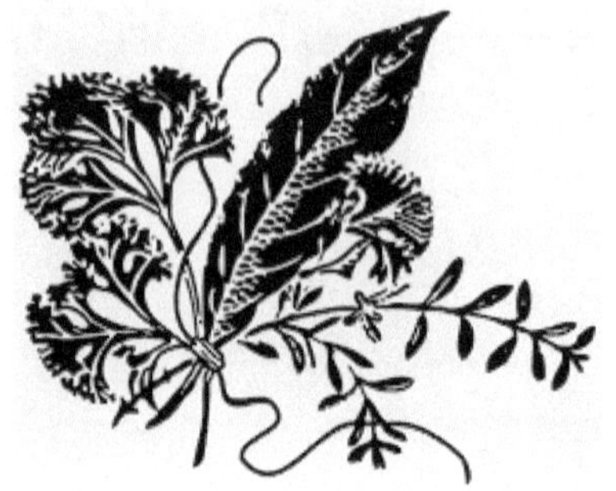

SCIATICA

(unresolved anger, suppressed fear, sadness)

Ginger poultice to warm up

The distressed area

Drinking celery juice helps alleviate

The pain

A change of cold and hot compresses

Helps reduce the pain severity

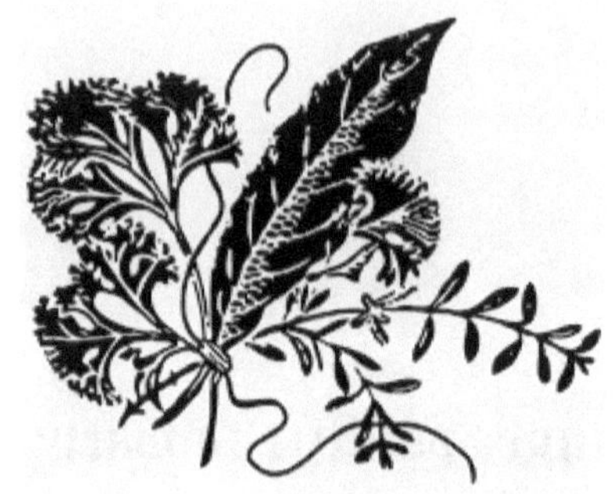

MAKING POULTICE

Make a cotton cloth or gauze of the size

Suitable to cover the affected area

Sprinkle a little of olive oil onto

The cloth and put the required herbs

On top of it

Wrap around the affected area

And secure

MAKING INFUSION

Put the required herbs in the pot

And pour hot water over it

Enough to cover the herbs

Leave the herbs in the pot for about

15 minutes and then

Strain the infusion into a cup

MAKING DECOCTION

Put the required herbs in the pot

With cold water and bring it to boil

Reduce heat and simmer for an hour

Let it cool and strain the liquid

into a cup

MAKING TINCTURE

Put the required herbs in a glass jar

Pour half vodka and half water over them

Store in a cool place for 2 weeks

Then strain into a wine press

Press the mixture through the wine press

Into a jug

Pour the strained liquid into

A clean dark glass

My great grandmother always used to tell me that you can help

People treat their symptoms but you cannot heal the problem

Unless they realize the emotional origin and cause

Every physical affliction starts with an emotional stress or trauma

She told me that most physical problems begin in one's mind

And if someone does not resolve his emotions in a timely

Manner, the affliction will persist by developing into a

Physical illness

As Dr. Francis Collins once said that

Genetics loads the gun, and the environment (lifestyle) pulls the trigger

She also said that one cannot heal in the place of pain, trying to relive and run the same emotions and feelings connected

To the traumatic situation

You have to change everything

For everything to change

Forgiveness alone can cleanse your lymphatic system by disposing of negative emotions as you choose to heal

Did you know that the emotion of Love is physically healing? It decreases cell death in one's body and reduces inflammation

Did you know that your gut cells renew themselves every

3-5 days? Your liver cells regenerate every 6 weeks, and

A new pathway in your brain can be established within

21 days if you decide to change your negative way of

Thought and take a different more positive direction.

I know and understand that some of us have a hard time

Of letting go

It is not easy to forgive someone when you

Feel they have done you wrong

However, illness has a different outlook when it comes to teaching us life lessons

When someone's words or actions may be compared to a

Snake's bite, your anger and resentment is the venom

You keep taking every day, compromising your own

Emotional well-being and physical condition

Forgive and let go That is the best thing you can do for yourself

And your children, for they too see and feel your pain.

Remember - you are not the only one, who needs to move on...

The end

www.ingramcontent.com/pod-product-compliance
Lightning Source LLC
Chambersburg PA
CBHW051056250726
48656CB00001B/324